HIGH FIBER FOOD LIST

The Complete Ingredient list and Food to Avoid For High Fiber Diet

Harley W. Norman

Table of Contents

Introduction

Are You Tired of Feeling Sluggish and Out of Sync? Could a Simple Change in Your Diet Transform Your Life?

In a bustling city where quick meals often mean unhealthy choices, Sarah felt trapped in a cycle of poor digestion, erratic energy levels, and frustrating weight fluctuations. Like many of us, she searched for a solution that didn't involve restrictive diets that were impossible to follow. Then, she discovered the transformative power of something surprisingly simple: fiber.

"High Fiber Food List" wasn't just a book for Sarah; it was a new beginning. Through its pages, she learned that incorporating more fiber-rich foods into her meals could revitalize her health in ways she never imagined.

The benefits unfolded as she turned each page:

- **Improved Digestion:** No more bloating or discomfort after meals, just a smooth, functioning digestive system.
- **Steady Energy Levels:** She waved goodbye to the mid-afternoon crashes that had her reaching for sugary snacks.
- **Enhanced Weight Management:** Fiber's filling nature meant fewer cravings and more effective weight control.

- **Reduced Risk of Chronic Diseases:** A fiber-rich diet supports heart health and helps in managing blood sugar levels, protecting against diabetes and heart disease.

But Sarah, like many potential readers, had her doubts. Would this book be another complex diet plan, difficult to understand and follow? Absolutely not.

Managing Objections:
- **Simplicity:** "High Fiber Food List" breaks down complex nutritional information into easy, actionable steps. It's not about overhauling your diet overnight but making small, impactful changes.
- **Variety:** Afraid of eating bland and boring meals? The book offers a rich variety of delicious, fiber-rich recipes that keep your taste buds happy and your health in check.
- **Practicality:** With tips on how to read food labels, integrate fiber at every meal, and adjust fiber intake for every family member, this guide is tailored for real life.
- **Support:** Understand that adjustments to your diet can bring about physical changes. The book addresses how to manage common side effects of increasing fiber in your diet, such as gas and bloating, with proven strategies that work.

Sarah's story is a testimony to the life-altering benefits of making better food choices. "High Fiber Food List" is more than just a book; it's a partner in your journey towards a healthier life. Why wait to feel better, have more energy, and embrace a healthier lifestyle?

Transform your health, one fiber-rich meal at a time. Discover how the smallest changes can make the biggest impact. Your journey to a revitalized, vibrant life starts here.

The Importance of Fiber in the Diet

Fiber is a crucial component of a healthy diet, often overlooked in favor of more immediate nutritional concerns like protein or vitamins. However, its role in maintaining various aspects of health makes it indispensable. Found primarily in fruits, vegetables, whole grains, and legumes, fiber offers multiple health benefits including digestive health, weight management, and disease prevention.

One of the primary benefits of fiber is its ability to aid digestion. It does this by adding bulk to the stool, which helps to keep the digestive system clean and moving efficiently. This not only helps to prevent constipation but also aids in the smooth operation of the gut, which can prevent the discomfort of bloating and gas. Additionally, a diet rich in fiber can foster a healthy gut microbiome, which is crucial for overall health, aiding in everything from immune system function to mental health.

Beyond digestion, fiber plays a key role in weight management. High-fiber foods are more filling than their low-fiber counterparts, which can help to reduce overall calorie intake by making people feel satiated sooner and for longer periods. This feeling of fullness can help to curb overeating and snacking, which is crucial for weight control and obesity prevention.

Fiber also has important implications for chronic disease management and prevention. For instance, soluble fiber, which dissolves in water to form a gel-like substance, can help to lower blood cholesterol levels and stabilize blood glucose levels. This can reduce the risk of heart disease and help manage diabetes. Furthermore, studies have shown that a high-fiber diet may reduce the risk of developing certain types of cancer, including colon cancer. The mechanisms behind this protective effect include fiber's ability to speed up the elimination of waste through the digestive system, thereby reducing the gut's exposure to potential carcinogens.

Moreover, incorporating a variety of high-fiber foods from the "High Fiber Food List" into the diet ensures that one not only benefits from the fiber itself but also from the array of other nutrients that these foods offer. For example, fruits like berries are rich in antioxidants in addition to fiber, and legumes are good sources of protein and iron. This synergy of nutrients can further enhance the health benefits of a high-fiber diet.

In essence, the significance of fiber in the diet extends beyond basic digestive health. It encompasses vital aspects of health maintenance, from aiding in weight management to preventing chronic diseases. A diverse, fiber-rich diet not only supports physical health but also contributes to overall well-being, making fiber an essential component of a balanced diet.

Understanding Fiber: Soluble vs. Insoluble

Fiber is a key component of a healthy diet, essential for digestive health and overall wellness. It is classified into two types: soluble and insoluble, each with distinct benefits and sources. Understanding the differences between these two types of fiber is crucial for implementing a balanced high-fiber diet.

Soluble fiber dissolves in water to form a gel-like substance that can help lower blood cholesterol and glucose levels. This type of fiber is particularly effective in regulating the body's use of sugars, helping to control blood sugar levels and reduce the spike in insulin that typically follows a meal. Foods rich in soluble fiber include oats, peas, beans, apples, citrus fruits, carrots, barley, and psyllium.

On the other hand, insoluble fiber does not dissolve in water. It is found in the seeds and skins of fruit as well as in whole grains and vegetables. Insoluble fiber helps add bulk to the stool and appears to help food pass more quickly through the stomach and intestines, which helps prevent or alleviate constipation. Common sources of insoluble fiber are whole wheat flour, wheat bran, nuts, beans, cauliflower, green beans, and potatoes.

Both types of fiber are vital for health, yet they serve different purposes within the digestive system. A diet rich in both soluble and insoluble fiber can prevent a variety of health issues such as constipation, irritable bowel syndrome, and diverticulitis. Moreover, a high-fiber diet can also help in weight management by making meals feel more filling, thus often reducing the amount of food eaten.

For those looking to enhance their diet with more fiber, it is important to gradually increase intake to give the body time to adjust. This gradual approach helps manage the physical responses such as bloating or gas that some experience when they suddenly increase their fiber intake. Drinking plenty of water is also essential, as it helps fiber move through the digestive system more easily, reducing the potential for discomfort.

Incorporating a balance of both types of fiber into meals not only supports digestive health but also contributes to overall well-being, making fiber a critical component of a healthy diet. Understanding the roles and sources of soluble and insoluble fiber can empower individuals to make informed choices about their food, leading to better health outcomes and a more balanced approach to eating.

The Benefits of a High-Fiber Diet

Digestive Health

Fiber plays a crucial role in maintaining digestive health, an essential part of overall wellness, especially when combined with high-protein foods. A diet rich in both fiber and protein supports the digestive system in several ways, enhancing gut function and contributing to a more balanced and healthful eating pattern.

High-fiber foods help to keep the digestive system clean and efficient. By absorbing water, fiber increases the softness and bulk of the stool, making it easier to pass and reducing the likelihood of constipation. This regularity is key for the quick and effective elimination of waste and toxins from the body. Additionally, fiber-rich foods such as vegetables, fruits, whole grains, and legumes feed the beneficial bacteria in the gut. These bacteria are crucial for gut health, aiding in digestion and the absorption of nutrients, and they also play a role in strengthening the immune system.

Protein, an essential macronutrient found in meats, dairy products, nuts, and beans, complements a high-fiber diet by providing the necessary components for enzyme production and muscle repair, which are vital for a healthy digestive tract. Proteins are also involved in hormone synthesis, many of which regulate digestion and metabolism.

When combined, a diet that is high in both fiber and protein can help mitigate common digestive issues such as irritable bowel syndrome (IBS) and inflammatory bowel disease (IBD). The fiber component helps reduce symptoms by improving consistency and regularity of bowel movements, while protein supports the healing and maintenance of the gut lining.

Furthermore, a balanced intake of fiber and protein can help manage and prevent diverticular disease. High-fiber diets can decrease the pressure in the colon, thereby reducing the risk of diverticular formation. Protein's role in tissue repair and maintenance further aids in preventing infections and promoting quick recovery from diverticulitis.

It is important to increase fiber intake gradually to avoid potential side effects such as bloating, gas, or discomfort. Drinking plenty of water is crucial as it facilitates the passage of fiber through the digestive system, making the process smoother and more effective.

By understanding the synergistic effects of fiber and protein in the diet, individuals can better manage their digestive health, leading to improved overall health and well-being. This holistic approach not only aids digestion but also supports other body functions, creating a strong foundation for a healthy lifestyle.

Blood Sugar Control

Maintaining stable blood sugar levels is a crucial aspect of managing overall health, particularly for those with diabetes or at risk of developing the condition. A diet high in fiber, especially when combined with good sources of protein, can significantly improve blood sugar control. This combination slows down the process of digestion, which in turn stabilizes blood sugar levels by preventing rapid spikes and crashes.

Fiber, particularly soluble fiber, has a notable impact on blood sugar levels. It forms a gel-like substance in the gut, which slows the absorption of sugars into the bloodstream. This slow absorption ensures that glucose enters the bloodstream gradually, leading to more stable blood sugar levels throughout the day. Foods like beans, oats, and some fruits are high in soluble fiber and are beneficial in a high-fiber, high-protein diet.

Protein also plays a vital role in blood sugar management by influencing the secretion of hormones like insulin, which helps manage blood glucose levels. Including a good protein source at each meal can help prevent the blood sugar peaks and valleys that can occur after eating high-carbohydrate foods. For instance, combining vegetables rich in fiber with lean meats, fish, or eggs—which provide high-quality protein—can be an effective strategy for enhancing blood sugar control.

Moreover, diets rich in both fiber and protein can lead to improved insulin sensitivity. This is particularly important for people with type 2 diabetes or those who are insulin resistant. Improved insulin sensitivity means the body is better able to use the insulin it produces or receives through medication, which further aids in blood sugar regulation.

Another benefit of a high-fiber, high-protein diet is that it can reduce the glycemic index of the overall meal. The glycemic index measures how quickly a food causes an increase in blood glucose levels; foods lower on this index are better for blood sugar control. By choosing low-glycemic index foods and enhancing these choices with fiber and protein, one can significantly improve their diet's impact on blood sugar levels.

Lastly, a diet that includes ample fiber and protein is generally more satisfying, which can prevent overeating. This is crucial for weight control, which is a significant factor in managing diabetes and enhancing blood sugar control. Being overweight can impair the body's ability to regulate glucose, so managing weight through diet can have a profound impact on overall health.

Incorporating these elements into one's diet not only supports blood sugar control but also contributes to a healthier lifestyle that can prevent the onset of diabetes and other related health issues. With mindful choices and an understanding of the synergistic effects of fiber and protein, individuals can take significant steps towards maintaining optimal health.

Heart Health

A high-fiber diet is widely recognized for its positive effects on heart health. Fiber, particularly soluble fiber found in many fruits, vegetables, and whole grains, plays a crucial role in reducing blood cholesterol levels, a key factor in the prevention of cardiovascular disease. Soluble fiber does this by binding with cholesterol particles in the digestive system and moving them out of the body before they're absorbed. Regular consumption of high-fiber foods can lead to a significant reduction in total and low-density lipoprotein (LDL) cholesterol, commonly referred to as "bad" cholesterol. This decrease in LDL cholesterol reduces the risk of forming plaques in the arteries, which can lead to atherosclerosis, heart attacks, and strokes.

In addition to lowering cholesterol, a high-fiber diet also benefits heart health by aiding in weight management. Obesity is a significant risk factor for cardiovascular disease. Fiber-rich foods are generally more filling than low-fiber foods, which can help control appetite and prevent overeating. This can lead to weight loss or help maintain a healthy weight, reducing the burden on the heart and lowering the risk of heart disease.

Fiber also has beneficial effects on blood pressure. Several studies have shown that diets high in fiber are associated with lower blood pressure. High blood pressure is another major risk factor for heart disease, as it forces the heart to work harder to pump blood through the body, which can weaken the heart over time and lead to poor heart function.

Furthermore, fiber can improve insulin sensitivity by slowing the absorption of sugar, helping to control blood sugar levels. Improved insulin sensitivity reduces the risk of metabolic syndrome, a cluster of conditions that includes increased blood pressure, high blood sugar, excess body fat around the waist, and abnormal cholesterol levels. Metabolic syndrome increases the risk for heart disease, stroke, and diabetes.

A diet rich in high-fiber foods is not only good for the heart but also contributes to overall health. For those looking to improve heart health through diet, incorporating a variety of fiber-rich foods into daily meals can be a practical and effective strategy. This might include choosing whole grains over refined grain products, opting for fruits and vegetables with edible skins, and including a variety of legumes in the diet. As with any dietary change, it is important to increase fiber intake gradually to allow the body time to adjust, and to ensure adequate fluid intake to help fiber function effectively in the body.

Weight Management

Fiber plays a pivotal role in weight management, which is often overlooked in discussions focused primarily on protein and caloric intake. A high-fiber diet contributes to weight control through several mechanisms, enhancing the effectiveness of a high-protein food regimen.

Fiber's primary benefit for weight management is its ability to increase feelings of fullness. Foods high in fiber, such as fruits, vegetables, whole grains, and legumes, take longer to eat and digest. This slow digestion process means that fiber-rich meals stay in the stomach longer, prolonging the sensation of fullness and reducing overall appetite. As a result, individuals on high-fiber diets tend to eat fewer calories without experiencing constant hunger.

In addition to increasing satiety, fiber helps regulate blood sugar levels, which can be particularly important for weight management. By slowing the absorption of sugar, high-fiber foods prevent insulin spikes that can lead to increased fat storage and hunger pangs. Stable blood sugar levels contribute to longer periods of satiety and diminish the desire for snacking between meals, which is a common obstacle in weight management.

Fiber also has a relatively low calorie content, which means adding fiber to the diet can increase food volume without significantly increasing caloric intake. This is crucial for those looking to lose weight or maintain a healthy weight without feeling deprived. By incorporating more high-fiber foods into meals, individuals can enjoy larger, more satisfying portions while still adhering to a calorie-controlled diet.

The synergy between high-fiber and high-protein foods can be particularly effective for weight loss and maintenance. Protein also promotes satiety and, when combined with fiber, can lead to even greater effects on fullness and appetite control. For instance, a meal that includes lean proteins like chicken or fish along with fiber-rich foods such as a quinoa salad or a side of steamed broccoli provides a balanced, nutrient-dense meal that can help manage weight effectively.

Moreover, a diet high in both fiber and protein can enhance metabolic health. Fiber can improve digestive health and aid in the elimination of waste, which can improve overall metabolic efficiency. A well-functioning digestive system is essential for weight management, as it helps the body process and eliminate unnecessary waste more effectively.

For those aiming to manage their weight, gradually increasing fiber intake while maintaining adequate protein intake can ensure that the body adjusts without discomfort, such as bloating or gas, which can sometimes accompany a sudden increase in fiber. Drinking plenty of water with high-fiber foods is essential to help the fiber move through the digestive tract and prevent any digestive discomfort.

Overall, incorporating high-fiber foods into a high-protein diet offers a multifaceted approach to weight management. It not only aids in controlling appetite and calorie intake but also supports metabolic processes that are crucial for maintaining a healthy weight.

Preventing Certain Cancers

A high-fiber diet is widely recognized for its many health benefits, including the potential to reduce the risk of developing several types of cancer, particularly colorectal cancer. The mechanisms through which fiber contributes to cancer prevention are multi-faceted and involve both the physical properties of fiber and its effects on body processes.

Fiber increases the bulk of the stool and accelerates the passage of food through the digestive tract. This means that carcinogens, substances in food that can cause cancer, have less time to come into contact with the intestinal walls. Additionally, fiber fermentation in the large intestine produces short-chain fatty acids that are thought to nourish colon cells and potentially inhibit cancerous growths.

Evidence suggests that diets rich in fiber reduce the risk of colorectal cancer and possibly other forms of cancer, such as breast cancer. High-fiber foods can help to maintain a healthy weight, as they are more filling and tend to be lower in calories. This is crucial since excess body weight is a recognized risk factor for various cancers, including breast, prostate, lung, colon, and kidney cancers.

Moreover, fiber helps to regulate blood sugar levels and reduce insulin spikes, which is significant because high levels of insulin and insulin-like growth factor-1 (IGF-1) have been linked to some cancers. Stable insulin levels help to reduce inflammation, another risk factor for cancer.

While the focus on high fiber aligns with preventive strategies against cancer, it is also important to consider the overall quality of the diet. A diet that includes a variety of fruits, vegetables, whole grains, and legumes, all high in fiber, provides numerous phytochemicals and nutrients that contribute to reduced cancer risk.

By adopting a diet that includes high-fiber foods, individuals not only support their digestive health but also adopt a powerful ally in the fight against cancer. The protective effects of fiber, combined with a healthy lifestyle that includes physical activity and avoiding smoking, create a comprehensive approach to cancer prevention.

Comprehensive Guide to High-Fiber Foods

Vegetables

Vegetable	Fiber Content (per serving)	Serving Size	Cooking Method	Cooking Time	Nutritional Highlights
Broccoli	5.1g	1 cup chopped	Steam	5 minutes	Rich in vitamin C, vitamin K, iron
Spinach	4.3g	1 cup cooked	Sauté	2 minutes	High in vitamin A, vitamin C, calcium
Carrots	3.6g	1 cup chopped	Boil	4 minutes	Good source of beta-carotene, vitamin K

Vegetable	Fiber Content (per serving)	Serving Size	Cooking Method	Cooking Time	Nutritional Highlights
Brussels Sprouts	4.0g	1 cup halved	Roast	20 minutes	Contains antioxidants, vitamin K, vitamin C
Sweet Potatoes	4.0g	1 medium	Bake	45 minutes	High in vitamin A, vitamin B6
Kale	2.6g	1 cup chopped	Steam	5 minutes	Rich in vitamins A, C, K, and minerals
Artichokes	6.9g	1 medium	Boil	25 minutes	Good source of magnesium, vitamin C
Peas	8.8g	1 cup	Boil	3 minutes	High in protein, vitamins A, C, K

Vegetable	Fiber Content (per serving)	Serving Size	Cooking Method	Cooking Time	Nutritional Highlights
Acorn Squash	9.0g	1 cup baked	Bake	60 minutes	Provides vitamin C, B vitamins
Green Beans	2.7g	1 cup	Steam	5 minutes	Contains vitamin K, vitamin C, manganese
Collard Greens	5.0g	1 cup cooked	Sauté	10 minutes	High in calcium and vitamin A
Turnips	3.1g	1 cup chopped	Boil	10 minutes	Good source of vitamin C
Butternut Squash	2.8g	1 cup cubed	Roast	30 minutes	High in vitamin A, potassium
Beets	3.8g	1 cup	Roast	45 minutes	Provides folate, manganese

Vegetable	Fiber Content (per serving)	Serving Size	Cooking Method	Cooking Time	Nutritional Highlights
Zucchini	1.2g	1 cup sliced	Sauté	7 minutes	Low in calories, high in potassium
Parsnips	5.6g	1 cup slices	Roast	25 minutes	Rich in fiber, vitamin C, folate
Cauliflower	2.5g	1 cup chopped	Steam	5 minutes	Low in calories, high in vitamins C and K
Asparagus	2.8g	1 cup	Grill	10 minutes	Good source of vitamins A, C, E, K
Fennel	3.1g	1 cup sliced	Sauté	5 minutes	Provides vitamin C, potassium, manganese
Radishes	1.9g	1 cup sliced	Raw	0 minutes	Low calorie, high in

Vegetable	Fiber Content (per serving)	Serving Size	Cooking Method	Cooking Time	Nutritional Highlights
					vitamin C

This table is an excellent resource for anyone looking to diversify their dietary fiber sources through vegetables. Each vegetable listed provides a substantial amount of fiber, along with a unique blend of vitamins and minerals that support overall health. The cooking methods and times are also optimized to preserve the nutritional integrity of the vegetables.

Fruits

Fruit	Fiber (grams) per Serving	Serving Size	Instructions	Cooking Time
Apple	4.4	1 medium (3" diameter)	Eat raw or add to salads; great for baking.	Raw/Bake: 30 min
Banana	3.1	1 medium	Peel and eat or blend into smoothies.	Raw
Orange	3.1	1 medium	Peel and eat or juice.	Raw
Strawberries	3.0	1 cup (halves)	Eat raw, add to cereals or desserts.	Raw
Raspberries	8.0	1 cup	Perfect for raw snacks or as a topping.	Raw

Fruit	Fiber (grams) per Serving	Serving Size	Instructions	Cooking Time
Blueberries	3.6	1 cup	Eat raw or use in smoothies and baking.	Raw/Bake: 15 min
Pear	5.5	1 medium	Eat raw, add to salads, or poach.	Raw/Poach: 20 min
Peach	2.0	1 medium	Eat raw or grill.	Raw/Grill: 10 min
Blackberries	7.6	1 cup	Eat raw or use in desserts and sauces.	Raw
Plum	1.4	1 medium	Eat raw or use in desserts.	Raw
Mango	2.6	1 cup (slices)	Peel and eat raw or blend into	Raw

Fruit	Fiber (grams) per Serving	Serving Size	Instructions	Cooking Time
			smoothies.	
Guava	8.9	1 cup (slices)	Eat raw or use in smoothies and salads.	Raw
Kiwi	2.1	1 large	Peel and eat or add to fruit salads.	Raw
Cherries	3.2	1 cup	Eat raw or use in pies and desserts.	Raw/Bake: 30 min
Pineapple	2.3	1 cup (chunks)	Eat raw, grill, or use in baking.	Raw/Grill: 10 min
Papaya	2.5	1 cup (cubes)	Eat raw or blend into tropical smoothies.	Raw

Fruit	Fiber (grams) per Serving	Serving Size	Instructions	Cooking Time
Apricot	1.0	1 medium	Eat raw or add to stews and cereal.	Raw/Stew: 45 min
Figs	1.9	1 medium	Eat raw, dried, or use in baking.	Raw/Bake: 15 min
Pomegranate	7.0	1 cup (seeds)	Eat seeds raw or sprinkle over salads.	Raw
Grapefruit	1.6	½ medium	Eat raw, add to salads, or use in smoothies.	Raw

Legumes

Legumes are a cornerstone of a high-fiber diet, providing not only fiber but also a range of essential nutrients including protein, iron, folate, and magnesium.

Legume	Fiber (per serving)	Other Nutrients	Serving Size	Cooking Time (approx.)
Black Beans	15g	High in protein, iron	1 cup	60-90 mins
Lentils	16g	Rich in folate, manganese	1 cup	20-30 mins
Chickpeas	12.5g	Good source of protein, zinc	1 cup	90-120 mins
Kidney Beans	13.1g	High in vitamin K1, potassium	1 cup	60-90 mins
Navy Beans	19.1g	Rich in B vitamins, magnesium	1 cup	60-90 mins
Peas	8.8g	Good source of vitamin C,	1 cup	5-10 mins

Legume	Fiber (per serving)	Other Nutrients	Serving Size	Cooking Time (approx.)
		vitamin A		
Pinto Beans	15.4g	High in protein, iron	1 cup	90-120 mins
Soybeans	10g	Rich in protein, omega-3 fatty acids	1 cup	180 mins
White Beans	11.3g	High in calcium, iron	1 cup	60-90 mins
Adzuki Beans	17g	Rich in potassium, protein	1 cup	60-90 mins
Black-eyed Peas	11g	Good source of folate, calcium	1 cup	60 mins
Lima Beans	13.2g	High in manganese, folate	1 cup	60 mins
Mung Beans	15.4g	Rich in potassium, magnesium	1 cup	45 mins

Legume	Fiber (per serving)	Other Nutrients	Serving Size	Cooking Time (approx.)
Red Lentils	15.6g	High in protein, folate	1 cup	15-20 mins
Fava Beans	9.2g	Good source of lean protein, iron	1 cup	80-90 mins
Split Peas	16.3g	High in protein, dietary fiber	1 cup	30-60 mins
Garbanzo Beans	12.5g	Rich in iron, phosphate	1 cup	90-120 mins
Great Northern Beans	12.4g	Good source of iron, magnesium	1 cup	60-90 mins
Cannellini Beans	11g	High in calcium, magnesium	1 cup	90-120 mins
Butter Beans	5.5g	Rich in protein, potassium	1 cup	60-90 mins

Instructions for Cooking Legumes:

- **Preparation:** Rinse legumes thoroughly under cold water to remove any dirt or impurities.

- **Soaking:** For most dried beans (like kidney beans, navy beans, and black beans), soaking overnight in water helps to reduce cooking time and improve digestibility. Lentils and split peas do not require soaking.

- **Cooking:** After soaking, drain and transfer the legumes to a large pot, covering them with fresh water. Bring to a boil, then reduce heat and simmer until tender. Add more water if needed during cooking. Note that adding salt or acidic ingredients should be done towards the end of cooking to avoid toughening the legumes.

This comprehensive guide to legumes in your high-fiber food list will not only enhance your meals but also contribute to your overall health, helping to manage weight, reduce cholesterol levels, and even assist in controlling blood sugar levels.

Whole Grains

Whole Grain	Serving Size	Cooking Time	Cooking Instructions	Nutritional Information per Serving
Quinoa	1 cup	15-20 min	Rinse under cold water, then boil in 2 cups of water. Reduce to simmer, cover, and cook until tender.	222 calories, 8g protein, 5g fiber
Brown Rice	1 cup	45 min	Rinse lightly, boil in 2.5 cups of water, simmer covered until water is absorbed.	216 calories, 5g protein, 3.5g fiber
Oats	1 cup	10-20 min	Boil in 2 cups of water or milk, simmer and stir occasionally until creamy.	166 calories, 6g protein, 4g fiber
Buckwheat	1 cup	10-12 min	Boil in 2 cups of water, simmer until	155 calories, 6g protein, 5g

Whole Grain	Serving Size	Cooking Time	Cooking Instructions	Nutritional Information per Serving
			tender.	fiber
Bulgur	1 cup	12-15 min	Boil in 2 cups of water, cover, and let stand until water is absorbed.	151 calories, 6g protein, 8g fiber
Millet	1 cup	20-25 min	Toast lightly then boil in 2.5 cups of water, simmer covered until all water is absorbed.	207 calories, 6g protein, 2g fiber
Barley	1 cup	50-60 min	Rinse and boil in 3 cups of water, simmer covered until tender.	193 calories, 6g protein, 6g fiber
Amaranth	1 cup	20-25 min	Boil in 3 cups of water, simmer covered until water is absorbed.	251 calories, 9g protein, 5g fiber

Whole Grain	Serving Size	Cooking Time	Cooking Instructions	Nutritional Information per Serving
Sorghum	1 cup	50-60 min	Boil in 4 cups of water, simmer until tender, drain excess water.	632 calories, 21g protein, 12g fiber
Teff	1 cup	15-20 min	Boil in 3 cups of water, simmer until water is absorbed.	255 calories, 10g protein, 7g fiber
Spelt	1 cup	50-60 min	Rinse and boil in 3 cups of water, simmer until tender.	246 calories, 10.7g protein, 7.6g fiber
Farro	1 cup	30-35 min	Rinse and boil in 3 cups of water, reduce to simmer until tender.	200 calories, 8g protein, 7g fiber
Freekeh	1 cup	20-25 min	Boil in 2.5 cups of water, simmer covered until tender.	132 calories, 4.5g protein, 4g fiber
Wild Rice	1 cup	45-50 min	Boil in 4 cups of water, simmer covered until kernels	166 calories, 6.5g protein, 3g fiber

Whole Grain	Serving Size	Cooking Time	Cooking Instructions	Nutritional Information per Serving
			pop open.	
Rye Berries	1 cup	50-60 min	Boil in 3 cups of water, simmer covered until tender.	188 calories, 7g protein, 8g fiber
Kamut	1 cup	50-60 min	Soak overnight, then boil in 3 cups of water, simmer until tender.	227 calories, 9.8g protein, 7.4g fiber
Black Rice	1 cup	30-35 min	Rinse and boil in 2.5 cups of water, simmer covered until tender.	160 calories, 5g protein, 3g fiber
Fonio	1 cup	5 min	Boil in 2 cups of water, simmer for 1 minute, then let stand covered for 4 minutes.	170 calories, 2g protein, 0g fiber
Chia Seeds	1 tbsp	No cook	Soak in 1 cup of water or any liquid	58 calories, 2g protein, 4g

Whole Grain	Serving Size	Cooking Time	Cooking Instructions	Nutritional Information per Serving
			to form a gel, typically takes 30 minutes.	fiber
Flaxseeds	1 tbsp	No cook	Grind and add to smoothies, cereals, or yogurt. Drinking water with flax is important to aid digestion.	55 calories, 1.9g protein, 2.8g fiber

Nuts and Seeds

Ingredient	Fiber (g) per Serving	Serving Size	Calories per Serving	Protein (g) per Serving	Cooking Time	Recommended Uses
1. Almonds	3.5	1 oz (23 nuts)	164	6	None	Snacking, almond butter, baking
2. Chia Seeds	10.6	1 oz	138	4.7	None	Smoothies, puddings, yogurt toppings
3. Flaxseeds	2.8	1 tbsp	37	1.3	None	Baked goods, smoothies, salads
4. Walnuts	1.9	1 oz (14 halves)	185	4.3	None	Baked goods, salads, homemade trail mixes
5. Pumpkin	1.7	1 oz	158	8.5	None	Salads, granola,

Ingredient	Fiber (g) per Serving	Serving Size	Calories per Serving	Protein (g) per Serving	Cooking Time	Recommended Uses
Seeds						snacking
6. Sunflower Seeds	3.0	1 oz	164	5.5	None	Snacking, salads, bread toppings
7. Sesame Seeds	1.1	1 tbsp	52	1.6	None	Topping for bread, salads, sushi
8. Pecans	2.7	1 oz (about 19 halves)	196	2.6	None	Desserts, salads, snacking
9. Hemp Seeds	1.0	1 tbsp	55	3.2	None	Smoothies, salads, yogurt
10. Pine Nuts	1.0	1 oz	191	3.9	None	Pesto, salads, pasta dishes
11. Brazil Nuts	2.1	1 oz (6 nuts)	187	4.1	None	Snacking, homemade nut

Ingredient	Fiber (g) per Serving	Serving Size	Calories per Serving	Protein (g) per Serving	Cooking Time	Recommended Uses
						mixes, baking
12. Hazelnuts	2.7	1 oz (21 nuts)	178	4.2	None	Baked goods, salads, snacking
13. Pistachios	2.9	1 oz (49 nuts)	159	5.7	None	Snacking, salads, crushed topping for fish or lamb
14. Macadamia Nuts	2.4	1 oz (12 nuts)	204	2.2	None	Baked goods, crushed for seafood coatings
15. Cashews	0.9	1 oz (18 nuts)	157	5.1	None	Snacking, vegan cheese substitutes, sauces

Ingredient	Fiber (g) per Serving	Serving Size	Calories per Serving	Protein (g) per Serving	Cooking Time	Recommended Uses
16. Coconut (shredded)	2.5	1 oz	185	1.9	None	Baked goods, curry dishes, toppings
17. Millet Seeds	2.3	1 oz	106	3.1	20 min	Porridge, salads, side dishes
18. Quinoa Seeds	2.6	1 oz	111	4.0	15 min	Side dishes, salads, pilafs
19. Buckwheat Seeds	4.5	1 oz	103	3.8	15-20 min	Porridge, pancakes, gluten-free baking
20. Sorghum Seeds	3.3	1 oz	106	3.5	50-60 min	Salads, pilafs, popped as a snack

Foods to Limit or Avoid for Optimal Fiber Intake

Processed and Refined Foods

Processed/Refined Food	Reason to Avoid
White Bread	Stripped of its natural fiber during processing, white bread lacks the nutritional benefits of whole-grain alternatives.
Regular Pasta	Made from refined wheat, regular pasta has most of its fiber and nutrients removed during processing.
White Rice	Like white bread, white rice has had its fiber-rich outer husk removed, reducing its fiber content significantly.
Sugary Cereals	Often made with refined grains and high amounts of sugar, these cereals offer little nutritional value and minimal fiber.

Processed/Refined Food	Reason to Avoid
Potato Chips	High in calories and fats, potato chips are typically low in fiber and contribute to unhealthy weight gain.
Cookies	Made from refined flour and high in sugar and fats, cookies provide very little fiber and are calorie-dense.
Soda	Sugary sodas contribute to weight gain and provide no nutritional benefits or fiber.
Deli Meats	Processed meats are high in sodium and preservatives, offering little nutritional value and no fiber.
Frozen Dinners	Often high in sodium and additives, many frozen dinners are made with refined grains and lack sufficient fiber.
Candy	High in sugar and unhealthy fats, candy is devoid of fiber and nutrients.
Instant Noodles	These contain refined carbs, are high in sodium, and very low in fiber.
Packaged Snacks	Snack cakes, pastries, and other packaged goods are usually made with

Processed/Refined Food	Reason to Avoid
	refined grains and are low in fiber.
Fast Food Burgers	Typically made with white buns and processed ingredients, these are low in fiber and high in unhealthy fats.
Margarine	Often containing trans fats, which are harmful to heart health, margarine has no fiber and is best avoided.
Microwave Popcorn	Pre-packaged versions often contain unhealthy fats and are low in fiber compared to their natural counterparts.
Breakfast Sausages	Processed and high in fat, these often contain fillers that are low in fiber.
Fruit Snacks	Despite the name, these snacks often contain more sugar than fruit and very little fiber.
Store-bought Salad Dressings	High in sugar and preservatives, these dressings add calories without providing fiber.
Flavored Yogurts	Often high in added sugars and low in fiber, especially compared to plain

Processed/Refined Food	Reason to Avoid
	yogurts.
Canned Soups	High in sodium and often made with refined ingredients, canned soups generally offer little fiber.

Each of these foods not only contributes minimally to your daily fiber intake but also potentially hinders overall health due to high levels of sugars, unhealthy fats, and additives. Limiting these foods can help improve dietary quality and increase the intake of necessary nutrients, including fiber, vital for maintaining good health.

High Sugar Foods

When aiming to increase your dietary fiber intake, it's essential to be mindful of consuming high sugar foods. These foods can counteract some of the health benefits that high fiber foods offer, such as improved blood sugar control and weight management.

High Sugar Food	Reasons to Avoid
Soda	High in added sugars and empty calories, contributes to weight gain and provides no nutritional value or dietary fiber.
Candy	Loaded with sugar and often fats, very low in nutrients and fiber, can lead to energy spikes and crashes.
Baked goods (cakes, pies)	Often high in both sugar and unhealthy fats, low in fiber, contributes to poor glycemic control and weight gain.
Ice cream	High in sugar and fat, contributing to increased calorie intake and potential weight gain, very little to no fiber.
Sweetened yogurt	Contains added sugars that can significantly increase calorie intake; opt for plain and add fruit

High Sugar Food	Reasons to Avoid
	for fiber.
Cereal bars	Many contain high levels of sugar and low fiber, despite being marketed as healthy; read labels carefully.
Breakfast cereals	Often contain a high amount of added sugars; choosing whole grain, low sugar options is better for fiber intake.
Cookies	Provide excessive sugars and fats with minimal essential nutrients and almost no fiber.
Fruit juices	Lack the fiber of whole fruits and are high in sugar, which can lead to energy spikes and increased caloric intake.
Energy drinks	High in sugar and caffeine, can lead to spikes in insulin levels and have little nutritional value.
Condiments (like ketchup)	Can contain high amounts of hidden sugars, adding unnecessary calories without fiber or significant nutritional benefits.
Jam and jelly	High in sugar, lacking the fiber found in whole fruit; opt for natural or light versions where possible.

High Sugar Food	Reasons to Avoid
Dried fruit (sugared)	Often coated with additional sugar, reducing their nutritional quality compared to fresh or naturally dried fruits.
Processed snacks	High in refined sugars and unhealthy fats, low in fiber and other nutrients, contributing to poor health outcomes.
Flavored coffee drinks	High in syrups and sugars, can contain as much sugar as several candy bars, very low in dietary fiber.
Sports drinks	While marketed as healthy, they can be high in sugars and are only necessary for endurance athletes.
Sweetened canned fruits	The syrup in canned fruits is high in sugar, negating the fiber benefits of the fruit; choose fruit canned in water.
Barbecue sauce	High in sugar, significantly adding to caloric intake without beneficial nutrients or fiber.
Granola (sweetened)	Although it may contain oats and nuts, the high sugar content overshadows the potential fiber benefits.

High Sugar Food	Reasons to Avoid
Pastries	High in sugar and fat, they contribute to calorie excess and provide very little in terms of fiber or essential nutrients.

Reducing intake of these high sugar foods can significantly enhance the effectiveness of a high-fiber diet, supporting better digestive health, improved blood sugar control, and overall healthier eating patterns. By focusing on whole, fiber-rich foods, you can avoid the pitfalls of excessive sugar consumption and its associated health risks.

Low Fiber Vegetables and Fruits

Vegetable/Fruit	Fiber (grams) per Serving	Serving Size	Reasons to Limit/Avoid for High Fiber Diet
Iceberg Lettuce	0.5	1 cup, shredded	Low in fiber compared to darker, leafier greens like spinach.
Cucumbers	0.5	½ cup, sliced	Mostly water; minimal fiber content.
Celery	0.6	1 stalk	High water content, very low in fiber.
Zucchini	0.6	½ cup, sliced	Low fiber; other squashes offer more fiber.
White Potatoes	0.8 (without skin)	1 small	Much of the fiber is in the skin, which is often removed.
Pumpkin	0.6	½ cup, canned	Lower fiber content compared to other winter squashes.

Vegetable/Fruit	Fiber (grams) per Serving	Serving Size	Reasons to Limit/Avoid for High Fiber Diet
Onions	1.1	½ cup, chopped	Low in fiber, used more for flavor enhancement.
Green Peppers	1.0	½ cup, sliced	Lower fiber content compared to other vegetables.
Turnips	1.0	½ cup, cubes	Lower fiber content; other root vegetables have more fiber.
Cauliflower	1.0	½ cup, chopped	Relatively low in fiber compared to its cruciferous counterparts.
Sweet Corn	1.8	½ cup	Moderate in fiber, but there are higher fiber alternatives.
White Mushrooms	0.7	½ cup, sliced	Lower in fiber compared to other mushrooms.
Cantaloupe	0.9	1 cup, cubes	Mostly water and sugar with very low fiber.
Watermelon	0.4	1 cup, cubes	High water content, very low fiber.

Vegetable/Fruit	Fiber (grams) per Serving	Serving Size	Reasons to Limit/Avoid for High Fiber Diet
Honeydew Melon	0.8	1 cup, cubes	Low fiber content, though rich in vitamin C.
Peaches (canned)	0.6	½ cup	Often peeled and processed, reducing fiber content significantly.
Oranges (juice)	0.2	½ cup	Juice removes the fibrous pulp, reducing fiber intake.
Grapes	0.9	½ cup	Low fiber content relative to serving size.
Pineapple	0.5	½ cup, chunks	Relatively low in fiber for a fruit.
Cherry Tomatoes	0.7	½ cup	Lower fiber content compared to whole or sliced tomatoes.

For individuals focused on enhancing their fiber intake, selecting alternatives with higher fiber counts is recommended. This list helps to identify those fruits and vegetables which might be less beneficial in a high-fiber diet, encouraging choices that have a more substantial impact on digestive health and overall dietary fiber goals.

Refined Grains

Refined grains have undergone processing that removes the bran and germ, leading to a loss of natural fiber, vitamins, and minerals.

Refined Grain	Reasons to Avoid
White Rice	Lacks fiber, vitamins, and minerals found in brown rice. Increases blood sugar levels more rapidly.
White Bread	Low in fiber and nutrients due to the removal of the wheat kernel's outer layers. Often contains added sugars.
White Pasta	Made from refined white flour, which leads to a spike in blood sugar and lacks dietary fiber.
White Flour	Stripped of bran and germ, reducing its fiber and nutrient content significantly.
Instant Oatmeal	Often has added sugars and salt, and the oats have been finely cut to cook quickly, reducing their fiber.
Pretzels	Typically made with white flour, high in sodium and low in fiber.
Cornflakes	Highly processed, low in fiber, and often high in added sugars.

Refined Grain	Reasons to Avoid
Puffed Rice	Processed to remove fiber and often used in sugary cereals.
Rice Cakes	Made from white rice, low in fiber and can spike blood sugar levels.
Crackers	Usually made from refined flours, lacking in fiber and potentially high in fats and salt.
Bagels	Typically made with white flour, resulting in a high-calorie, low-fiber food.
Corn Tortillas	Often made from refined corn flour, lacking in fiber compared to whole grain versions.
Rice Noodles	Made from white rice flour and devoid of fiber, with a high glycemic index.
Couscous	Usually made from refined wheat flour, lacks the fiber of whole grain varieties.
Pizza Dough	Commercial varieties are often made from white flour, adding empty calories and minimal fiber.
Cake Flour	Highly refined and intended for soft-textured cakes, very low in fiber.
Croissants	Made from refined flour and high in butter, offering little nutritional benefit and low fiber.

Refined Grain	Reasons to Avoid
Breadcrumbs	Often made from white bread, containing low fiber and sometimes high in added sugars and fats.
Pancakes	Typically prepared with white flour, leading to low fiber content and often served with sugary syrups.
Waffles	Like pancakes, made from white flour and frequently topped with high-sugar additions.

Consuming refined grains can contribute to a number of health issues, such as weight gain, higher blood sugar levels, and an increased risk of chronic diseases. These grains are stripped of the most nutritious parts, reducing their beneficial properties and leaving behind simple carbohydrates that digest quickly. For a healthier diet, it's advisable to choose whole grains, which retain all the natural fiber, vitamins, and minerals, and offer numerous health benefits including better digestive health and a lower risk of heart disease and diabetes.

Incorporating High-Fiber Foods into Your Diet

Recipes and Meal Ideas

Integrating high-fiber foods into daily meals enhances not only digestive health but overall wellness. Starting the day with a breakfast of oatmeal topped with berries and chia seeds can provide a fiber-rich and nutrient-packed beginning. For added flavor and fiber, mix in some crushed nuts such as almonds or walnuts.

Lunch offers another great opportunity to boost fiber intake. A hearty vegetable soup with lentils or beans, served alongside a whole-grain bread, makes for a filling and nutritious midday meal. For those who prefer salads, mixing a variety of colorful vegetables like spinach, carrots, and bell peppers, topped with avocado slices and sprinkled with sunflower seeds, offers a delicious and fiber-dense option.

Snacks can be both satisfying and high in fiber. Raw vegetables such as carrot sticks, bell pepper slices, or broccoli florets dipped in hummus not only provide crunch but are also laden with fiber. Alternatively, an apple or pear can satisfy sweet cravings while boosting fiber consumption.

For dinner, experimenting with whole grains like quinoa or barley as side dishes can substantially increase fiber content. Pair these grains with grilled vegetables and a lean protein such as chicken or fish for a balanced and fiber-rich meal. For those looking to incorporate more plant-based proteins, trying a stir-fry with tofu and a variety of vegetables like snap peas, mushrooms, and bok choy can be both satisfying and high in fiber.

When it comes to desserts, opting for recipes that use fruits as the main ingredient can be a wise choice. Baked apples or pears, for instance, sprinkled with a bit of cinnamon and nutmeg, provide a sweet finish without compromising on fiber content. For a more indulgent yet fiber-rich dessert, a blackberry and raspberry crisp with a topping of rolled oats and whole wheat flour offers a delightful treat.

Overall, by choosing ingredients that are naturally high in fiber and combining them creatively across meals, maintaining a diet rich in this essential nutrient becomes both achievable and enjoyable.

Tips for Increasing Fiber Gradually

Increasing dietary fiber gradually is key to allowing the body to adjust without discomfort. Here are some practical tips for integrating more fiber into your diet effectively and comfortably.

Start by replacing refined grains with whole grains. Instead of white bread, pasta, or rice, opt for whole wheat bread, whole grain pasta, and brown or wild rice. These swaps are simple and can significantly boost your fiber intake.

Add legumes to your meals a few times a week. Beans, lentils, and chickpeas are high in fiber and can be incorporated into salads, soups, and casseroles. Start with small servings and increase gradually to avoid gastrointestinal discomfort.

Incorporate a variety of vegetables into every meal. Aim for at least half your plate to be vegetables. They can be raw, steamed, or lightly sautéed. Start by adding one extra serving of vegetables a day and increase as your digestive system adapts.

Snack on high-fiber foods. Replace chips and cookies with raw vegetables, nuts, seeds, or whole fruit. These foods not only increase fiber but also provide healthy fats and vitamins.

Increase your fruit intake, focusing on whole fruits rather than juices, which lack fiber. Berries, oranges, apples, and pears all have high fiber content and can be eaten as snacks or added to cereals and yogurt.

Be mindful of your breakfast choices. Start your day with a high-fiber breakfast cereal, oatmeal, or a smoothie with fruits, vegetables, and a spoonful of flaxseeds or chia seeds.

Stay hydrated. Increasing fiber without adequate water intake can lead to constipation. Drinking plenty of water helps fiber work better in your digestive system.

Listen to your body. Everyone's digestive system reacts differently to increased fiber. If you experience bloating or discomfort, slow down the increase and give your body time to adjust.

Use these tips to boost your fiber intake slowly and effectively, making your transition to a high-fiber diet smooth and beneficial for your overall health.

How to Read Food Labels for Fiber Content

Reading food labels is an essential skill for anyone looking to increase their dietary fiber intake. The nutrition facts label on packaged foods provides vital information about the fiber content per serving, helping individuals make informed choices that align with their health goals.

When examining a food label, the first step is to look at the serving size, which is usually listed at the top of the label. This amount determines how much of the food corresponds to the nutritional values provided, including fiber. It's important to compare this to the actual amount you consume. If you eat double the serving size listed, you will need to double the nutritional values, including the fiber content.

The next step is to check the total carbohydrate section of the label, where dietary fiber is listed under this category. The amount of fiber is given in grams and sometimes as a percentage of the Daily Value (DV). The DV is a guide to the nutrients in one serving of food and is based on a daily intake of 2,000 calories. For dietary fiber, a DV of 25 grams is used as a reference. Foods with 5 grams of fiber or more per serving are considered high in fiber, whereas those with less than 3 grams are considered low.

Also, be wary of terms like "multigrain," "stone-ground," "100% wheat," or "bran," which are often used to make products appear healthier. These terms do not necessarily mean that the product is high in fiber. Instead, look for words like "whole grain" or "whole wheat" as the first ingredient on the ingredients list. Whole grain products include all parts of the grain, providing more fiber than refined grains.

Moreover, it's important to be cautious about added sugars and artificial ingredients that might be present even in high-fiber foods. Some manufacturers add extra sugar to compensate for the altered texture and taste when fiber is added to products. Therefore, scanning the ingredients list for added sugars and opting for products with natural ingredients and without added sugars is beneficial.

Lastly, while increasing fiber intake, it's essential to do so gradually and increase water intake as well. This helps manage the body's adjustment to higher fiber levels and prevents digestive discomfort, such as bloating and gas.

By understanding how to read and interpret food labels accurately, you can choose high-fiber foods more wisely, which is a crucial step in enhancing your diet and improving your overall health. This skill not only helps in achieving a high-fiber diet but also empowers you to make dietary choices that can lead to long-term health benefits.

Breakfast

Breakfast Item	Ingredients	Instructions	Nutritional Information (per serving)	Serving Size	Cooking Time
Oatmeal with Berries	Rolled oats, mixed berries, honey, chia seeds	Cook oats, top with berries and chia seeds, drizzle with honey	8g fiber, 250 calories	1 bowl	10 min
Chia Pudding	Chia seeds, almond milk, vanilla extract, maple syrup	Mix ingredients, refrigerate overnight	10g fiber, 200 calories	1 cup	5 min + overnight
Whole Wheat	Whole wheat flour,	Mix ingredients,	5g fiber, 150 calories	2 pancak	20 min

Breakfast Item	Ingredients	Instructions	Nutritional Information (per serving)	Serving Size	Cooking Time
Pancakes	eggs, milk, baking powder	cook on griddle		es	
Avocado Toast	Whole grain bread, avocado, lime, salt, pepper	Mash avocado, spread on toasted bread	6g fiber, 220 calories	1 slice	5 min
Bran Muffins	Wheat bran, whole wheat flour, honey, milk, eggs	Mix ingredients, bake in muffin tins	7g fiber, 180 calories	1 muffin	25 min
High-Fiber Smoothie	Spinach, banana, pear, flaxseeds, almond	Blend all ingredients until smooth	9g fiber, 210 calories	1 glass	5 min

Breakfast Item	Ingredients	Instructions	Nutritional Information (per serving)	Serving Size	Cooking Time
	milk				
Veggie Omelette	Eggs, spinach, mushrooms, onions, cheese	Cook vegetables, add beaten eggs, fold omelette	4g fiber, 300 calories	1 omelette	15 min
Quinoa Breakfast Bowl	Quinoa, almond milk, cinnamon, nuts, dried fruit	Cook quinoa in almond milk, add toppings	8g fiber, 320 calories	1 bowl	20 min
Apple Cinnamon Overnight Oats	Rolled oats, diced apples, cinnamon,	Mix ingredients, refrigerate overnight	7g fiber, 250 calories	1 jar	5 min + overnight

Breakfast Item	Ingredients	Instructions	Nutritional Information (per serving)	Serving Size	Cooking Time
	yogurt, honey				
Breakfast Burrito	Whole wheat tortilla, scrambled eggs, beans, salsa	Wrap ingredients in tortilla, serve	12g fiber, 350 calories	1 burrito	10 min
Muesli	Rolled oats, nuts, seeds, dried fruits, yogurt	Mix ingredients, serve with yogurt	6g fiber, 230 calories	1 cup	5 min
Nutty Banana Bread	Whole wheat flour, bananas, walnuts, eggs, honey	Bake mixture in loaf pan	5g fiber, 210 calories	1 slice	60 min

Breakfast Item	Ingredients	Instructions	Nutritional Information (per serving)	Serving Size	Cooking Time
Sweet Potato Hash	Sweet potatoes, onions, bell peppers, eggs	Cook vegetables, crack eggs into pan, cover to cook eggs	7g fiber, 290 calories	1 plate	25 min
Pear and Walnut Salad	Sliced pears, walnuts, mixed greens, vinaigrette	Toss ingredients with dressing	5g fiber, 180 calories	1 bowl	10 min
Pumpkin Porridge	Pumpkin puree, oats, cinnamon, nutmeg, almond milk	Cook all ingredients together	10g fiber, 240 calories	1 bowl	15 min

Breakfast Item	Ingredients	Instructions	Nutritional Information (per serving)	Serving Size	Cooking Time
Berry Yogurt Parfait	Greek yogurt, granola, mixed berries, honey	Layer ingredients in a glass	6g fiber, 230 calories	1 glass	5 min
Mediterranean Frittata	Eggs, spinach, tomatoes, feta cheese, onions	Mix ingredients, bake in oven	4g fiber, 260 calories	1 slice	35 min
Cottage Cheese and Fruit Plate	Cottage cheese, mixed fresh fruit, nuts	Arrange cottage cheese, fruit, and nuts on plate	4g fiber, 200 calories	1 plate	5 min

Breakfast Item	Ingredients	Instructions	Nutritional Information (per serving)	Serving Size	Cooking Time
Spiced Lentil Breakfast Patties	Lentils, breadcrumbs, spices, eggs	Form patties and pan fry	8g fiber, 250 calories	2 patties	30 min
Fig and Ricotta Toast	Whole grain bread, ricotta cheese, fresh figs, honey	Spread ricotta on toasted bread, top with sliced figs and honey	5g fiber, 200 calories	1 slice	5 min

This table is designed to make it easy to incorporate high-fiber ingredients into traditional and creative breakfast dishes. Whether you prefer a quick and easy smoothie or a hearty burrito, each option packs a nutritious punch that will keep you feeling full and energized throughout the morning.

Lunch

Recipe Name	Ingredients	Instructions	Nutritional Information (per serving)	Serving Size	Cooking Time
Quinoa Veggie Bowl	Quinoa, black beans, avocado, cherry tomatoes, spinach, lime, olive oil	Cook quinoa. Mix with beans, veggies, and dressing. Serve topped with sliced avocado.	Calories: 350, Fiber: 9g	1 bowl	25 min
Chickpea Salad Sandwich	Chickpeas, whole grain bread, celery, Greek	Mash chickpeas and mix with yogurt, mustard,	Calories: 400, Fiber: 8g	1 sandwich	15 min

Recipe Name	Ingredients	Instructions	Nutritional Information (per serving)	Serving Size	Cooking Time
	yogurt, mustard, lettuce	and celery. Serve on bread with lettuce.			
Lentil Soup	Lentils, carrots, onions, celery, tomatoes, garlic, vegetable broth	Sauté veggies, add lentils and broth, simmer until lentils are tender.	Calories: 300, Fiber: 12g	1 bowl	45 min
Black Bean Tacos	Black beans, corn tortillas, salsa, lettuce, cheese,	Warm beans and tortillas, assemble tacos with toppings.	Calories: 380, Fiber: 11g	2 tacos	20 min

Recipe Name	Ingredients	Instructions	Nutritional Information (per serving)	Serving Size	Cooking Time
	lime				
Broccoli Almond Salad	Broccoli, almonds, dried cranberries, yogurt dressing	Combine all ingredients and toss with dressing.	Calories: 280, Fiber: 5g	1 cup	10 min
Veggie Stir-Fry	Bell peppers, snap peas, carrots, tofu, brown rice, soy sauce	Stir-fry veggies and tofu, serve over rice.	Calories: 410, Fiber: 6g	1 bowl	30 min

Recipe Name	Ingredients	Instructions	Nutritional Information (per serving)	Serving Size	Cooking Time
Spinach and Feta Wrap	Whole wheat tortillas, spinach, feta cheese, eggs, onions	Sauté onions, add eggs and spinach, wrap in tortilla with feta.	Calories: 290, Fiber: 4g	1 wrap	15 min
Sweet Potato Chili	Sweet potatoes, kidney beans, tomatoes, onion, chili spices	Cook all ingredients until potatoes are tender and chili is thick.	Calories: 460, Fiber: 13g	1 bowl	40 min
Mediterranean Farro Salad	Farro, cucumbers, olives, feta, tomatoes,	Cook farro, mix with chopped veggies and	Calories: 330, Fiber: 8g	1 bowl	30 min

Recipe Name	Ingredients	Instructions	Nutritional Information (per serving)	Serving Size	Cooking Time
	red onion, vinaigrette	feta, dress with vinaigrette.			
Butternut Squash Soup	Butternut squash, onions, vegetable stock, nutmeg, cream	Roast squash, blend with sautéed onions and stock, simmer, add cream.	Calories: 250, Fiber: 7g	1 bowl	1 hr
Avocado Toast	Whole grain bread, avocado, radishes, sesame seeds, lime	Toast bread, top with mashed avocado, sliced radishes, and sesame	Calories: 310, Fiber: 10g	1 slice	10 min

Recipe Name	Ingredients	Instructions	Nutritional Information (per serving)	Serving Size	Cooking Time
		seeds.			
Barley and Veggie Salad	Barley, cherry tomatoes, cucumber, parsley, lemon dressing	Cook barley, mix with veggies and dressing.	Calories: 290, Fiber: 9g	1 bowl	40 min
Baked Falafel Wrap	Chickpeas, whole wheat tortillas, lettuce, tahini sauce, garlic	Blend chickpeas with spices, bake into falafel, wrap with veggies and tahini.	Calories: 360, Fiber: 11g	1 wrap	30 min

Recipe Name	Ingredients	Instructions	Nutritional Information (per serving)	Serving Size	Cooking Time
Beet and Goat Cheese Salad	Beets, goat cheese, walnuts, arugula, balsamic glaze	Roast beets, slice and mix with arugula, cheese, nuts, and drizzle with glaze.	Calories: 280, Fiber: 6g	1 plate	45 min
Hummus and Veggie Plate	Hummus, carrot sticks, cucumber slices, bell peppers, whole grain pita	Serve hummus with sliced veggies and pita for dipping.	Calories: 270, Fiber: 8g	1 plate	10 min
Mushroom Risotto	Arborio rice,	Cook rice with	Calories: 410, Fiber:	1 bowl	45 min

Recipe Name	Ingredients	Instructions	Nutritional Information (per serving)	Serving Size	Cooking Time
	mushrooms, Parmesan cheese, chicken stock, onions	sautéed mushrooms and onions in stock, finish with cheese.	3g		
Pesto Pasta Salad	Whole wheat pasta, pesto, sun-dried tomatoes, pine nuts, spinach	Cook pasta, mix with pesto, tomatoes, nuts, and fresh spinach.	Calories: 380, Fiber: 7g	1 bowl	20 min
Tuna Salad on Rye	Canned tuna, rye bread, lettuce,	Mix tuna with mayo, celery, and lemon,	Calories: 340, Fiber: 5g	1 sandwich	10 min

Recipe Name	Ingredients	Instructions	Nutritional Information (per serving)	Serving Size	Cooking Time
	mayo, celery, lemon juice	serve on rye with lettuce.			
Roasted Vegetable Panini	Zucchini, bell peppers, onion, whole grain bread, mozzarella	Roast vegetables, assemble panini with cheese, grill until crispy.	Calories: 420, Fiber: 6g	1 sandwich	25 min
Tomato Basil Soup	Tomatoes, basil, garlic, onion, vegetable stock, olive	Sauté garlic and onion, add tomatoes and stock, blend until	Calories: 180, Fiber: 4g	1 bowl	30 min

Recipe Name	Ingredients	Instructions	Nutritional Information (per serving)	Serving Size	Cooking Time
	oil	smooth, simmer with basil.			

This collection of recipes demonstrates that high-fiber lunches can be diverse, flavorful, and fulfilling. Whether you're in the mood for a hearty bowl of chili, a refreshing salad, or a satisfying sandwich, there's a high-fiber option to suit every palate while contributing to a healthy, fiber-rich diet.

Recipe Name	Ingredients	Instructions	Nutritional Information	Serving Size	Cooking Time
Quinoa & Black Bean Salad	Quinoa, black beans, tomatoes, avocado, lime, cilantro, olive oil	Cook quinoa, mix with other ingredients, dress with lime & oil	300 calories, 15g fiber	1 bowl	30 min
Chickpea Vegetable Stew	Chickpeas, carrots, tomatoes, spinach, onions, garlic, spices	Sauté veggies, add chickpeas and spices, simmer	250 calories, 12g fiber	1 bowl	45 min
Lentil Soup	Lentils, carrots, celery, onion,	Cook lentils with veggies and broth until tender	220 calories, 16g fiber	1 bowl	1 hr

Recipe Name	Ingredients	Instructions	Nutritional Information	Serving Size	Cooking Time
	garlic, broth, herbs				
Barley & Mushroom Risotto	Barley, mushrooms, onions, garlic, broth, Parmesan	Cook barley in broth, add mushrooms, finish with Parmesan	350 calories, 8g fiber	1 serving	50 min
Whole Wheat Pasta Primavera	Whole wheat pasta, bell peppers, zucchini, tomato sauce	Boil pasta, sauté vegetables, combine with sauce	330 calories, 10g fiber	1 plate	30 min
Baked Sweet Potato with Lentils	Sweet potatoes, lentils, onions, garlic,	Bake sweet potatoes, cook lentils with spices, serve	400 calories, 13g fiber	1 serving	1 hr 20 min

Recipe Name	Ingredients	Instructions	Nutritional Information	Serving Size	Cooking Time
	cumin, yogurt	together			
Vegetable Stir Fry with Tofu	Tofu, broccoli, bell pepper, soy sauce, ginger, garlic	Sauté tofu, add vegetables and sauce, stir fry	270 calories, 11g fiber	1 plate	20 min
Butternut Squash Soup	Butternut squash, onions, garlic, broth, cream	Roast squash, blend with sautéed onions and broth, add cream	210 calories, 9g fiber	1 bowl	1 hr
Spicy Black Bean Tacos	Black beans, corn tortillas, avocado, salsa,	Warm beans and tortillas, assemble tacos	320 calories, 11g fiber	2 tacos	15 min

Recipe Name	Ingredients	Instructions	Nutritional Information	Serving Size	Cooking Time
	lettuce, cheese				
Broccoli and Cheddar Bake	Broccoli, cheddar cheese, whole wheat bread crumbs, eggs, milk	Mix ingredients, bake until golden	290 calories, 6g fiber	1 serving	35 min
Moroccan Chickpea Stew	Chickpeas, sweet potatoes, tomatoes, spices, onions	Sauté onions, add ingredients, simmer	360 calories, 14g fiber	1 bowl	40 min
Spinach and Feta Stuffed Chicken	Chicken breasts, spinach, feta, onions, garlic	Stuff chicken with sautéed spinach and feta, bake	310 calories, 4g fiber	1 serving	45 min

Recipe Name	Ingredients	Instructions	Nutritional Information	Serving Size	Cooking Time
Eggplant Parmesan	Eggplant, marinara sauce, mozzarella, Parmesan, breadcrumbs	Layer fried eggplant with sauce and cheeses, bake	350 calories, 7g fiber	1 serving	1 hr
Cauliflower Curry	Cauliflower, coconut milk, curry paste, chickpeas, spinach	Sauté cauliflower, add coconut milk and curry, simmer	300 calories, 10g fiber	1 bowl	40 min
Stuffed Bell Peppers	Bell peppers, quinoa, black beans, corn, cheese, spices	Stuff peppers with quinoa mix, bake	380 calories, 9g fiber	1 pepper	1 hr

Recipe Name	Ingredients	Instructions	Nutritional Information	Serving Size	Cooking Time
Zucchini Lasagna	Zucchini, ricotta, marinara sauce, mozzarella, ground turkey	Layer ingredients, replacing pasta with sliced zucchini, bake	320 calories, 8g fiber	1 serving	1 hr 10 min
Bean and Barley Soup	Barley, kidney beans, tomatoes, celery, carrots, broth	Cook barley and beans with veggies and broth	270 calories, 14g fiber	1 bowl	1 hr
Mushroom and Spinach Polenta	Polenta, mushrooms, spinach, Parmesan, garlic	Cook polenta, sauté veggies, serve together	310 calories, 5g fiber	1 serving	30 min

Recipe Name	Ingredients	Instructions	Nutritional Information	Serving Size	Cooking Time
Vegan Chili	Kidney beans, black beans, tomatoes, corn, vegan meat substitute	Cook all ingredients together to blend flavors	280 calories, 13g fiber	1 bowl	50 min
Apple Walnut Salad	Mixed greens, apples, walnuts, blue cheese, vinaigrette	Combine ingredients, dress with vinaigrette	250 calories, 5g fiber	1 bowl	10 min

These recipes offer a variety of flavors and are packed with nutrients to help maintain a healthy, fiber-rich diet. Each meal is designed to provide a fulfilling and tasty option that supports digestive health and contributes to overall wellness.

Snack	Ingredients	Instructions	Nutritional Information	Serving Size	Cooking Time
Apple Peanut Butter Slices	Apple, peanut butter	Slice apple, spread peanut butter on slices	Fiber: 4g, Calories: 150	1 apple	No cook
Chia Seed Pudding	Chia seeds, almond milk, honey	Mix ingredients, refrigerate overnight	Fiber: 10g, Calories: 200	1 cup	8 hours (rest)
Oatmeal Energy Balls	Rolled oats, peanut butter, honey	Mix ingredients, form balls, chill	Fiber: 3g, Calories: 100 per ball	2 balls	30 min (chill)
Veggie Sticks with	Carrot, celery, hummus	Cut veggies, serve with hummus	Fiber: 5g, Calories: 150	1 cup veggies	No cook

Snack	Ingredients	Instructions	Nutritional Information	Serving Size	Cooking Time
Hummus					
Raspberries with Yogurt	Raspberries, Greek yogurt	Top yogurt with raspberries	Fiber: 4g, Calories: 90	1 cup	No cook
Almond Date Bars	Dates, almonds, oats	Process ingredients, press into bars, chill	Fiber: 6g, Calories: 180 per bar	1 bar	1 hour (chill)
Roasted Chickpeas	Chickpeas, olive oil, seasoning	Roast chickpeas with oil and spices	Fiber: 6g, Calories: 150 per serving	1/2 cup	30 min
Banana Oat Cookies	Bananas, oats	Mash bananas, mix with oats, bake	Fiber: 3g, Calories: 50 per cookie	2 cookies	15 min
Quinoa Salad	Quinoa, veggies,	Mix quinoa with	Fiber: 7g, Calories:	1 cup	15 min

Snack	Ingredients	Instructions	Nutritional Information	Serving Size	Cooking Time
Cups	vinaigrette	veggies, serve in lettuce	120 per cup		
Whole Wheat Pita with Avocado	Whole wheat pita, avocado, lemon juice	Mash avocado, spread on pita	Fiber: 6g, Calories: 200 per serving	1 pita	No cook
Pear with Almond Butter	Pear, almond butter	Slice pear, spread almond butter on slices	Fiber: 5g, Calories: 150	1 pear	No cook
Popcorn	Popcorn kernels, olive oil	Pop kernels in oil	Fiber: 4g, Calories: 100 per serving	3 cups popped	10 min
Nutty Banana Bread	Whole wheat flour,	Bake banana bread with	Fiber: 5g, Calories: 165 per	1 slice	1 hour

Snack	Ingredients	Instructions	Nutritional Information	Serving Size	Cooking Time
	bananas, nuts	nuts	slice		
Berry Smoothie	Mixed berries, spinach, almond milk	Blend ingredients	Fiber: 5g, Calories: 130	1 cup	5 min
Granola Trail Mix	Granola, nuts, dried fruit	Mix ingredients	Fiber: 4g, Calories: 150 per serving	1/2 cup	No cook
Stuffed Figs	Figs, goat cheese, walnuts	Stuff figs with cheese and nuts, bake	Fiber: 5g, Calories: 120 per fig	2 figs	15 min
Edamame	Edamame, sea salt	Boil edamame, sprinkle with salt	Fiber: 8g, Calories: 100 per serving	1 cup	5 min

Snack	Ingredients	Instructions	Nutritional Information	Serving Size	Cooking Time
Carrot Raisin Salad	Carrots, raisins, lemon juice, honey	Mix carrots with raisins and dressing	Fiber: 4g, Calories: 90 per serving	1 cup	No cook
Baked Apple Chips	Apples, cinnamon	Thinly slice apples, sprinkle with cinnamon, bake	Fiber: 4g, Calories: 50 per serving	1 cup	1 hour
Guacamole and Whole Wheat Crackers	Avocado, lime juice, salt, whole wheat crackers	Prepare guacamole, serve with crackers	Fiber: 5g, Calories: 180 per serving	1/4 cup guacamole	No cook

Dessert

Dessert	Ingredients	Instructions	Nutritional Information	Serving Size	Cooking Time
Apple Bran Muffins	Whole wheat flour, apple, wheat bran, cinnamon, honey	Mix ingredients, bake at 375°F	5g fiber, 150 calories	1 muffin	20 min
Chia Pudding	Chia seeds, almond milk, honey, vanilla extract	Combine ingredients, refrigerate overnight	10g fiber, 200 calories	1 cup	8 hrs (rest)
Oatmeal Banana Cookies	Bananas, oats, walnuts, cinnamon	Mash bananas, mix with oats, bake at 350°F	3g fiber, 100 calories	2 cookies	15 min
Raspberry Fiber	Raspberries, oats, whole	Layer ingredients,	4g fiber, 120 calories	1 bar	30 min

Dessert	Ingredients	Instructions	Nutritional Information	Serving Size	Cooking Time
Bars	wheat flour, honey	bake at 350°F			
Pear and Quinoa Crumble	Pear, quinoa, almonds, cinnamon, honey	Layer pears and quinoa, bake at 375°F	6g fiber, 210 calories	1 serving	45 min
Black Bean Brownies	Black beans, cocoa powder, sugar, eggs, vanilla	Blend beans, mix ingredients, bake at 350°F	7g fiber, 180 calories	1 brownie	25 min
Almond Fig Cake	Dried figs, almond flour, eggs, honey	Mix ingredients, bake at 350°F	5g fiber, 230 calories	1 slice	30 min
Pumpkin Oat Cookies	Pumpkin puree, oats, maple	Mix ingredients, drop on	3g fiber, 90 calories	3 cookies	20 min

Dessert	Ingredients	Instructions	Nutritional Information	Serving Size	Cooking Time
	syrup, spices	sheet, bake at 350°F			
Carrot Cake Oatmeal Bars	Carrots, oats, walnuts, cinnamon, honey	Mix ingredients, bake at 350°F	4g fiber, 130 calories	1 bar	30 min
Coconut Mango Bites	Mango, coconut flakes, dates, lime juice	Blend ingredients, form balls, chill	2g fiber, 50 calories	2 bites	10 min + chill
Avocado Chocolate Mousse	Avocado, cocoa powder, honey, vanilla	Blend all ingredients until smooth	6g fiber, 220 calories	1/2 cup	10 min
Blueberry Lemon Bars	Blueberries, whole wheat flour,	Mix crust, top with berries, bake	3g fiber, 150 calories	1 bar	35 min

Dessert	Ingredients	Instructions	Nutritional Information	Serving Size	Cooking Time
	lemon, oats	at 375°F			
Pear Ginger Scones	Pears, whole wheat flour, ginger, buttermilk	Mix ingredients, shape scones, bake at 400°F	4g fiber, 180 calories	1 scone	25 min
Date Walnut Pie	Dates, walnuts, whole wheat pie crust, eggs	Mix filling, pour into crust, bake at 350°F	5g fiber, 250 calories	1 slice	40 min
Prune and Almond Tart	Prunes, almonds, whole wheat flour, honey	Layer prunes and almonds, bake at 350°F	6g fiber, 240 calories	1 slice	30 min
Chocolate Hazelnut Truffles	Hazelnuts, dates, cocoa powder, vanilla	Process ingredients, form truffles, chill	3g fiber, 70 calories	2 truffles	15 min + chill

Dessert	Ingredients	Instructions	Nutritional Information	Serving Size	Cooking Time
	extract				
Apple Cinnamon Galette	Apples, whole wheat pastry, cinnamon, sugar	Arrange apples on pastry, fold, bake at 375°F	4g fiber, 200 calories	1 piece	45 min
Mixed Berry Cobbler	Mixed berries, whole wheat flour, oats, sugar	Layer berries, top with dough, bake at 375°F	5g fiber, 160 calories	1 serving	30 min
Plum Spelt Muffins	Plums, spelt flour, cinnamon, maple syrup	Mix ingredients, spoon into tins, bake at 375°F	3g fiber, 140 calories	1 muffin	20 min
Lemon Poppy Seed Loaf	Whole wheat flour, poppy	Mix ingredients, bake at	2g fiber, 180 calories	1 slice	50 min

Dessert	Ingredients	Instructions	Nutritional Information	Serving Size	Cooking Time
	seeds, lemon zest, yogurt	350°F			

These desserts not only satisfy sweet cravings but also contribute to your daily fiber intake, supporting digestion and overall health. By incorporating these high-fiber recipes into your routine, you can enjoy indulgent flavors without compromising on nutrition.

Special Considerations

Managing Fiber Intake with IBS

Managing fiber intake is a critical aspect of controlling symptoms for individuals with Irritable Bowel Syndrome (IBS). This condition, characterized by symptoms such as cramping, abdominal pain, bloating, gas, diarrhea, and constipation, can be significantly influenced by diet, particularly by the types of fiber consumed.

For those with IBS, soluble fiber is often recommended over insoluble fiber. Soluble fiber dissolves in water to form a gel-like substance in the digestive tract, which can help regulate the movement of food and waste. It tends to slow digestion and can help stabilize blood sugar levels by slowing the absorption of sugar. More importantly, it can reduce diarrhea by absorbing excess water in the bowel. Foods high in soluble fiber include oats, psyllium, apples, oranges, carrots, and flaxseeds.

On the other hand, insoluble fiber does not dissolve in water and adds bulk to the stool. While this is generally beneficial for regular bowel movements, it can cause problems for IBS sufferers, such as exacerbating diarrhea and abdominal discomfort. Common sources of insoluble fiber include whole grains, nuts, tomatoes, raisins, broccoli, and cabbage.

People with IBS are advised to manage their fiber intake carefully:

- Start Slow: Gradually increase fiber intake. A sudden increase can lead to gas, bloating, and cramps. It's important to give the digestive system time to adjust.

- Monitor Symptoms: Keeping a food diary can be helpful in tracking which foods exacerbate or alleviate IBS symptoms. This personal record can guide adjustments in dietary choices.

- Stay Hydrated: Drinking sufficient water is crucial when increasing fiber intake, as it helps fiber move smoothly through the digestive system and reduces the risk of constipation.

- Consider a Fiber Supplement: If it's challenging to get enough fiber from food alone, a soluble fiber supplement like psyllium can be a controlled way to increase fiber intake without adding too many insoluble fibers to the diet.

- Consult with a Dietitian: Since IBS symptoms can vary widely, working with a dietitian can help tailor dietary recommendations to fit individual needs.

Balancing the types of fiber and monitoring the overall intake can significantly impact the quality of life for someone with IBS. Adapting to a high-fiber diet requires thoughtful consideration of the types of fiber consumed and careful monitoring of their effects on symptoms. A nuanced approach, emphasizing gradual changes and personal adjustments, is often most effective in managing IBS through diet.

High Fiber Diet in Children

Ensuring children consume an adequate amount of fiber is essential for their overall health, digestive wellness, and for establishing healthy eating habits early in life. A high-fiber diet for children not only helps maintain bowel regularity but also plays a crucial role in preventing obesity by making meals more satisfying and less calorie-dense.

The recommended daily intake of fiber for children varies by age and sex. Generally, the guideline is that children should consume an amount of fiber equivalent to their age plus five grams per day. For instance, a four-year-old should have about nine grams of fiber each day. As children grow older, their fiber needs approach adult levels, roughly 25 grams for females and 31 grams for males per day, according to dietary guidelines.

Introducing fiber into a child's diet should be a gradual process to prevent digestive discomfort such as bloating, gas, or constipation, which can occur with sudden increases in fiber intake. It's also important to ensure that children drink plenty of fluids, as fiber works best when it absorbs water.

Incorporating fiber-rich foods into a child's diet can be fun and versatile. Whole fruits, vegetables, whole grain products, beans, and legumes are excellent sources of fiber. Creative ways to include these might involve adding fruit to breakfast cereal, using whole wheat bread for sandwiches, or mixing beans into ground meat dishes like tacos or spaghetti sauce.

Creating a balanced plate is key. For example, an ideal dinner plate might include a small portion of grilled chicken, a large serving of mixed vegetables, some brown rice, and a piece of fruit for dessert. Snacks can also be fiber-rich; options include apple slices with peanut butter, carrot sticks with hummus, or a small handful of nuts.

While increasing fiber is beneficial, it's important to watch for signs of too much fiber, which can lead to a decrease in appetite if the child feels too full to eat other necessary nutrients throughout the day. If a child is showing less interest in eating or is experiencing digestive issues, it may be wise to adjust fiber intake and consult a pediatrician.

Educating children on the importance of fiber in their diet can also help them make informed dietary choices as they grow. Discussing how fiber helps their digestive system function better or how it keeps them feeling full longer can empower them to choose high-fiber foods willingly.

Overall, a balanced approach to increasing fiber in a child's diet not only supports their current health but also sets the foundation for healthier dietary habits that can last a lifetime.

Adjustments for the Elderly

Adjusting the fiber intake for elderly individuals requires careful consideration due to the changes in digestive systems that occur with age. As people grow older, the digestive system becomes less efficient, and high fiber intake can either be very beneficial or lead to digestive discomfort depending on how it is managed. It is important for elderly individuals to incorporate fiber into their diet gradually to allow their bodies to adapt without causing side effects such as bloating, gas, or constipation.

The benefits of a high-fiber diet for the elderly include improved bowel function, which helps prevent constipation—a common issue in older adults. Fiber can also help manage blood sugar levels, reduce the risk of heart disease by lowering cholesterol, and aid in weight management by helping individuals feel fuller longer. However, it is essential to balance fiber intake with adequate fluid consumption, as fiber works best when it absorbs water.

When making dietary adjustments, it is crucial to focus on soluble fiber sources like oatmeal, nuts, beans, apples, and blueberries, which are easier on the stomach and help with nutrient absorption. Insoluble fiber sources like whole grains and vegetables are also important, but they should be introduced more slowly to avoid overwhelming the digestive system.

Elderly individuals often take multiple medications, and fiber can interfere with the absorption of some drugs. Therefore, it is important to manage the timing of fiber consumption to ensure that it does not coincide directly with medications that could be affected.

To facilitate the inclusion of fiber in an elderly person's diet, foods should be prepared in a way that makes them easy to chew and digest. Cooking vegetables until they are tender, choosing whole-grain products that are soft such as whole grain breads and cereals, and using natural purées like apple sauce as a fiber supplement can all be beneficial practices.

Finally, it's beneficial for elderly people to have regular dietary reviews with healthcare providers to tailor fiber intake according to their specific health needs and digestive capacity. This personalized approach ensures that the dietary fiber benefits their overall health without causing discomfort or other complications. This care in managing fiber intake supports not just digestive health but contributes broadly to the wellbeing and quality of life in elderly individuals.

Conclusion

The journey through the world of high-fiber foods is not merely a dietary change but a lifestyle adjustment that can lead to profound improvements in health. By emphasizing the inclusion of a variety of fiber-rich foods such as fruits, vegetables, legumes, and whole grains, this guide offers a path to enhanced digestion, improved blood sugar regulation, lower cholesterol levels, and sustainable weight management. These benefits, in turn, contribute to a reduced risk of developing chronic diseases like type 2 diabetes, heart disease, and certain types of cancer.

Embracing a high-fiber diet also encourages a more mindful approach to eating. It prompts individuals to consider the nutritional value of their food, leading to healthier choices overall. Additionally, the satiating nature of fiber-rich foods can lead to reduced calorie intake without the feeling of deprivation that often accompanies other dietary regimens. This makes a high-fiber diet not only beneficial for health but also sustainable over the long term.

Moreover, this guide has addressed potential challenges such as the initial digestive discomfort that can accompany an increase in fiber intake. By recommending a gradual increase in fiber and adequate hydration, the guide helps mitigate these effects, making the transition smoother and more comfortable.

Ultimately, the aim of adopting a high-fiber diet should be to foster a balanced, healthful eating pattern that can be maintained throughout life. As research continues to reveal, the benefits of dietary fiber extend far beyond the digestive system, influencing overall health and well-being in numerous positive ways. This makes the pursuit of a high-fiber diet a worthwhile endeavor for anyone looking to enhance their health and quality of life.